The lion's Mane Mushroom

H.-G. Saenger

The Book:

The Lion's Mane Mushroom : The Healing Mushroom for the Nerves" is a comprehensive guide to the miracle mushroom Lion's Mane, a superfood that is gradually gaining attention for its many health benefits. This book explores the Lion's Mane mushroom, its origins, uses and potential in a way that is accessible to everyone from the layperson to the health professional. It combines historical knowledge, scientific research and practical guidance to give readers a holistic understanding of this potent mushroom.

The Author:

H.-G. Saenger
passionate reader and
author with a wide range of interests,
lives since 2020 with his second wife
wife in Thailand.

The lion's Mane Mushroom

The Nerve Whisperer

by

H.-G. Saenger

Table of Contents:

Book Introduction:

„The Lion's Mane: The Medicinal Mushroom for Your Nerves" is a comprehensive guide to the wonder that is Lion's Mane mushroom, a superfood that has been gradually gaining attention for its multitude of health benefits. This book explores the Lion's Mane mushroom, its origins, its uses, and its potential in a way that is accessible to everyone, from the layman to the health professional. It combines historical knowledge, scientific research, and practical guidance to give readers a holistic understanding of this potent mushroom.

The Lion's Mane mushroom, known scientifically as Hericium Erinaceus, is a unique medicinal mushroom, notable for its cascading spines that resemble a lion's mane. It has a rich history in traditional Asian medicine, where it has been used for centuries to treat a variety of health issues. Recent scientific research has started to confirm many of these traditional uses, revealing that Lion's Mane may indeed have significant health benefits, especially in relation to neurological and mental health. This has led to a surge in interest in Lion's Mane and its potential uses.

This book begins with an introduction to Lion's Mane, explaining what it is and where it comes from. It delves into the fascinating history of Lion's Mane, tracing its use from ancient times to the present day. The third chapter gives readers an in-depth understanding of Lion's Mane, explaining its unique structure and how it is that this humble mushroom can have such potent effects on the human body.

The subsequent chapters look at the specific health benefits of Lion's Mane. This includes its potential role in neurological health, its potential benefits for mental health, its immune-boosting properties, and its potential role in heart health and cancer prevention and treatment. These chapters combine a review of the latest scientific research with practical advice on how to use Lion's Mane for these purposes.

The latter part of the book is devoted to practical aspects of Lion's Mane. This includes a guide to cultivating your own Lion's Mane mushrooms, complete with step-by-step instructions and tips for success. There is also a chapter devoted to cooking with Lion's Mane, which includes a range of delicious and healthy recipes that allow readers to incorporate Lion's Mane into their diet in a tasty way.

As the author himself suffers from polyneuropathy in the lower extremities, he subjected himself to a self-experiment, which ultimately led to the writing of this book. The self-experiment is still ongoing, but the first results give him more than hope that there will be an improvement in his living conditions with regard to the previous limitations and pain caused by this disease. Apparently, the medicinal mushroom actually has a positive effect on the regeneration of the damaged nerve endings.

The book concludes with a look at the future of Lion's Mane, exploring ongoing research into its potential uses and the directions that this research may take in the future. This makes it a must-read for anyone interested in natural health, superfoods, or the fascinating world of medicinal mushrooms. Please note, writing full chapters for each of these topics would.

Chapter 1: Introduction to Lion's Mane Mushroom

The world of fungi holds many wonders, and among them, the Lion's Mane mushroom stands out for its striking appearance and intriguing health benefits. Known scientifically as Hericium erinaceus, this mushroom derives its common name from the unique structure of cascading spines that resemble the mane of a lion.

This chapter serves as an introduction to this fascinating organism, its natural habitat, its physical characteristics, its life cycle, and the various names it is known by around the world.

The Lion's Mane mushroom, belonging to the tooth fungus group, can be found in North America, Europe, and Asia. It grows on hardwoods, particularly on dead and dying trees, symbolizing nature's magnificent cycle of life, death, and rebirth. Often, these mushrooms are discovered by foragers in late summer and fall, clinging to logs and stumps in the woods, their pure white tendrils hanging down like a waterfall of icicles.

The fruiting body of the Lion's Mane mushroom is quite distinctive. It forms clusters of long spines - the ‚teeth' - that hang from a branched stem. These spines, or ‚icicles', produce the spores that allow the mushroom to reproduce. When young, the mushroom is often pure white and as soft as marshmallow, but as it ages, it can turn yellowish and become more brittle.

In culinary terms, Lion's Mane is considered a delicacy in many cultures. Its taste is often likened to seafood, similar to crab or lobster, and it retains a pleasant, meaty texture when cooked. It is used in a variety of dishes, including stir-fries, soups, and even tea. However, its value extends far beyond the kitchen.

Lion's Mane holds a special place in traditional medicine, particularly in China and Japan, where it has been used for centuries for its healing properties. These ancient cultures believed that the Lion's Mane mushroom could support gut health, boost the immune system, and even enhance brain function.

The Lion's Mane mushroom goes by many names, reflecting its global reach and the respect it commands. In Japan, it's known as „Yamabushitake," named after the Yamabushi monks who were believed to have used the mushroom for its cognitive benefits. In China, it's called „Hóu Tóu Gū," meaning monkey head mushroom, a nod to its unique appearance. In the West, apart from Lion's Mane, it's also known as bearded tooth mushroom or pom pom mushroom.

As we continue our journey through this book, we'll delve deeper into the Lion's Mane mushroom's medicinal properties, supported by modern scientific research. We'll explore how this unique fungus can support our neurological health, mental wellbeing, and overall immune system. Furthermore, we'll look at how we can incorporate Lion's Mane into our everyday lives, from cooking and eating this delicious mushroom to growing it in our homes.

The world of Lion's Mane is as fascinating as it is beneficial, and this journey promises to be an enlightening one. As we uncover the mysteries of this magnificent mushroom, we may find that it holds the key to many health benefits that modern society needs. So let us embark on this journey of discovery, understanding, and ultimately, better health through the power of Lion's Mane mushroom.

Chapter 2: History and Origin of Lion's Mane

Lion's Mane mushroom, or Hericium erinaceus, has a rich and fascinating history that spans continents and centuries. This chapter delves into the origin of this extraordinary mushroom, its early use in traditional medicine, and its journey to becoming a recognized superfood in the modern world.

While the exact origin of Lion's Mane mushroom is difficult to pinpoint, it is known to grow naturally in the temperate regions of North America, Europe, and Asia. This broad geographical distribution allowed various cultures to discover and utilize Lion's Mane independently, adding unique perspectives to its medicinal and culinary use.

In ancient China, Lion's Mane was highly regarded for its health-enhancing properties. The mushroom was often depicted in Chinese art and literature, symbolizing longevity and spiritual potency. The ancient Chinese medical text, the „Compendium of Materia Medica," written by Li Shizhen in the 16th century, lists Lion's Mane as a tonic for the five internal organs, a treatment for digestive ailments, and a cure for general weakness.

Similarly, in Japan, Lion's Mane, known as Yamabushitake, was used by the Yamabushis - hermit monks who practiced a form of mountain asceticism. It is said that these monks consumed Lion's Mane to maintain their vigor during their rigorous physical and spiritual practices. They also believed that the mushroom could enhance their cognitive abilities, aiding in their meditative practices.

In Europe, the Lion's Mane mushroom was less recognized for its medicinal properties but was highly prized for its culinary value. Its unique texture and flavor, reminiscent of seafood, made it a sought-after delicacy. It often featured in the traditional cuisine of Eastern Europe and was considered a special treat when it could be found in the wild.

As for the Native American tribes, while there isn't clear documentation, it is likely that they were aware of the Lion's Mane mushroom and its benefits, given their extensive knowledge of local flora and fauna.

Fast forward to the 20th century, with the advent of modern science and the ability to study organisms at a cellular level, interest in the Lion's Mane mushroom was rekindled. Scientific research began to explore the numerous health claims associated with Lion's Mane, focusing particularly on its potential neurological benefits.

This led to an increased global awareness of Lion's Mane, its recognition as a „smart" mushroom, and its inclusion in the list of natural „nootropics" - substances that can enhance cognitive function. Today, it is not uncommon to find Lion's Mane in various forms, from dietary supplements to gourmet dishes, reflecting its widespread acceptance and use.

In conclusion, the Lion's Mane mushroom has a long and storied history that crosses cultural and geographical boundaries. Its journey from a woodland curiosity to a recognized superfood is a testament to its unique properties and the human desire for natural health solutions. As we move forward, it is clear that the Lion's Mane mushroom will continue to play a vital role in our pursuit of optimal health and wellbeing.

Chapter 3: The Lion's Mane: Anatomy of a Superfood

To truly appreciate the power of the Lion's Mane mushroom, it's essential to understand its anatomy and the biochemical constituents that lend it its superfood status. This chapter will delve into the physical structure of Lion's Mane, its chemical composition, and the key compounds responsible for its health benefits.

The Lion's Mane mushroom, Hericium erinaceus, belongs to the tooth fungus group, so named for their distinctive tooth-like structures from which spores are released. The fruiting body of Lion's Mane is composed of cascading, icicle-like spines hanging from a branched or singular stem. These spines or ‚teeth' are where the spores that facilitate reproduction are produced. However, the true magic of Lion's Mane lies beneath its captivating exterior, in the complex array of bioactive compounds it houses. These compounds, primarily polysaccharides, terpenoids, sterols, and proteins, work in concert to give Lion's Mane its superfood status.

Among the polysaccharides are beta-glucans, complex sugars recognized for their immune-modulating properties. Beta-glucans interact with immune cells, bolstering the body's defenses against illness and disease. This explains Lion's Mane's long-standing use in traditional medicine as an immune booster.

But the two compounds that have attracted the most attention from the scientific community are hericenones and erinacines. These compounds, found respectively in the fruiting body and mycelium of the Lion's Mane mushroom, are potent stimulators of nerve growth factor (NGF) production.

NGF is a protein essential for the growth, maintenance, and survival of nerve cells, including neurons. It plays a crucial role in cognitive functions such as memory and learning. The ability of Lion's Mane to boost NGF production is the basis for its use as a natural nootropic and its potential in managing neurodegenerative disorders.

Other compounds present in Lion's Mane include antioxidants that help combat oxidative stress, a major contributor to aging and numerous diseases. Additionally, the mushroom contains several essential amino acids, minerals, and vitamins, further enhancing its nutritional profile.

Cultivating Lion's Mane under optimal conditions can also lead to the production of other beneficial compounds. For instance, when grown on a substrate containing brown rice, Lion's Mane has been found to produce erinacerins, another group of compounds with potential neuroprotective properties.

In conclusion, the Lion's Mane mushroom is more than just its impressive appearance. It's a powerhouse of bioactive compounds, each contributing to the mushroom's overall health benefits. Its unique combination of immune-modulating, neuroprotective, and antioxidant properties rightfully earns Lion's Mane its place as a superfood. As research continues to uncover the secrets housed within its majestic mane, the future of Lion's Mane in health and wellness appears promising.

Chapter 4: Understanding the Science Behind Lion's Mane

The science behind the Lion's Mane mushroom is as fascinating as it is promising. With an increasing number of studies exploring its potential health benefits, our understanding of this unique fungus continues to grow. This chapter aims to delve deeper into the scientific evidence supporting the health-promoting properties of Lion's Mane.

Neuroprotection and Cognitive Enhancement:

The most researched aspect of Lion's Mane is its impact on brain health. The mushroom's unique compounds, hericenones, and erinacines, stimulate the production of nerve growth factor (NGF), a protein crucial for the growth and maintenance of neurons. This has significant implications for neurodegenerative diseases such as Alzheimer's and Parkinson's. In preclinical studies, Lion's Mane has shown potential in slowing disease progression, reducing symptoms, and improving quality of life in these conditions.

Further, research suggests that Lion's Mane may enhance cognitive function. A 2009 study on older adults with mild cognitive impairment found that those who consumed Lion's Mane extract for 16 weeks showed significantly improved scores on cognitive function scales compared to a placebo group.

Mental Health Support:

Emerging research suggests that Lion's Mane may also offer benefits for mental health. Its ability to stimulate NGF production could help in the maintenance of a healthy mood, and preliminary studies have shown potential benefits in reducing symptoms of anxiety and depression.

Immune System Enhancement:

Lion's Mane contains beta-glucans, polysaccharides known for their immune-modulating properties. These compounds can stimulate the body's immune response, enhancing its ability to fend off pathogens. Animal studies have demonstrated that Lion's Mane can increase the activity of macrophages and other immune cells, indicating a more robust immune response.

Antioxidant Properties:

The presence of potent antioxidants in Lion's Mane helps combat oxidative stress, a primary contributor to aging and various chronic diseases. By neutralizing harmful free radicals, these antioxidants may offer protective effects against various health conditions, including heart disease and cancer.

Potential Anti-Cancer Properties:

Preliminary research suggests that Lion's Mane may have potential anti-cancer properties. In vitro and animal studies have shown that the mushroom can inhibit the growth and spread of certain types of cancer cells, including those of the liver, colon, gastric, and breast cancers. However, these promising results need confirmation in human studies.

While the scientific exploration of Lion's Mane is ongoing, the evidence so far offers a promising outlook on the potential health benefits of this mushroom. Its unique blend of bioactive compounds and their various effects on the human body make Lion's Mane a fascinating subject in the realm of natural health. As our understanding deepens, it becomes increasingly clear that the Lion's Mane mushroom has much to offer, not only for our current health but also as a potential preventative measure against various conditions.

Chapter 5: Lion's Mane and Neurological Health

The neurological benefits of Lion's Mane are perhaps its most fascinating aspect. Its unique ability to stimulate nerve growth factor (NGF) production sets it apart from most other known natural substances, offering significant potential in the realm of neurological health. This chapter will delve into Lion's Mane's effects on the nervous system, its potential in managing neurodegenerative diseases, and its role in cognitive enhancement.

Nerve Growth Factor and Neurogenesis:

Nerve Growth Factor is a protein essential for the growth, maintenance, and survival of neurons. It plays a crucial role in neurogenesis - the process of forming new neurons, which is critical for maintaining healthy cognitive function. The hericenones and erinacines in Lion's Mane stimulate NGF production, thereby promoting neurogenesis and potentially slowing or reversing neuronal damage.

Lion's Mane and Neurodegenerative Diseases:

Neurodegenerative diseases like Alzheimer's and Parkinson's are characterized by progressive neuronal loss. Current research suggests that Lion's Mane, with its ability to stimulate NGF production, could play a role in managing these diseases. Preclinical studies have shown that Lion's Mane extracts can reduce symptoms and slow disease progression in models of Alzheimer's and Parkinson's diseases. While human studies are still limited, these findings provide a promising foundation for future research.

Cognitive Enhancement:

The role of Lion's Mane in cognitive enhancement is backed by both traditional use and modern scientific research. The mushroom's ability to stimulate NGF production can support various cognitive functions, including memory, learning, and concentration. A clinical study on older adults with mild cognitive impairment showed that daily consumption of Lion's Mane led to significant cognitive improvement over a period of 16 weeks.

Lion's Mane and Mood Disorders:

Emerging research suggests that Lion's Mane may also support mental health. Anxiety and depression are linked to changes in brain structure and function, and the neurotrophic effects of Lion's Mane could potentially help manage these conditions. Preliminary studies indicate that Lion's Mane may help reduce symptoms of anxiety and depression, but further research is needed to fully understand these effects.

Neuroprotection:

Beyond its potential therapeutic uses, Lion's Mane could also offer neuroprotective benefits. By promoting neurogenesis and providing antioxidant support, Lion's Mane may help protect the nervous system from damage, potentially reducing the risk of neurological disorders.

In conclusion, the Lion's Mane mushroom's potential in promoting neurological health is impressive. While further research, particularly human clinical trials, is needed to fully understand its therapeutic potential, current evidence positions Lion's Mane as a promising natural ally in maintaining a healthy, well-functioning nervous system.

Chapter 6: Lion's Mane in Mental Health Support

Mental health disorders are a growing concern worldwide, and natural remedies like Lion's Mane are gaining attention for their potential role in mental health support. This chapter will explore the emerging evidence of Lion's Mane's potential benefits for mental health, including anxiety, depression, and mood regulation.

Lion's Mane and Anxiety:

Anxiety disorders are among the most common mental health issues, characterized by excessive worry and fear. Preliminary research indicates that Lion's Mane may help manage anxiety symptoms. In a study involving women with a variety of health complaints, including anxiety, taking Lion's Mane cookies for a month led to reduced feelings of irritation and anxiety. The exact mechanism is still under investigation, but it may involve the mushroom's ability to stimulate nerve growth factor and support a healthy stress response.

Lion's Mane and Depression:

Depression is a debilitating condition that affects millions worldwide. It is associated with changes in brain structure and function, particularly in areas responsible for mood regulation. As Lion's Mane can stimulate nerve growth factor and promote neurogenesis, it is thought that it may help counter these changes and thereby alleviate depressive symptoms. Indeed, early research, such as the study on women mentioned above, suggests that Lion's Mane can reduce depressive symptoms, although more research is needed to confirm these findings.

Lion's Mane and Cognitive Function:

Cognitive function plays a crucial role in mental health. Impaired memory, difficulty concentrating, and reduced ability to think clearly can significantly impact a person's quality of life and are common features of various mental health disorders. By promoting neurogenesis and supporting the health of neurons, Lion's Mane may help enhance cognitive function, potentially improving these aspects of mental health.

Lion's Mane and Stress:

Chronic stress is a risk factor for various mental health conditions, including anxiety and depression. It's thought that the adaptogenic properties of Lion's Mane may help the body better cope with stress, thereby reducing its impact on mental health. While specific research on Lion's Mane and stress is limited, its ability to support a healthy stress response could make it a valuable tool in mental health support.

In conclusion, while research on Lion's Mane's potential in mental health support is still in its early stages, preliminary findings are promising. Its unique neurotrophic effects, combined with its potential mood-regulating and stress-relieving properties, suggest that Lion's Mane may offer valuable support for mental health. However, it's essential to remember that while Lion's Mane may help support mental health, it should not replace professional medical advice or treatment. Mental health disorders are serious conditions that require appropriate medical attention.

- 22 -

Chapter 7: Immune Boosting Properties of Lion's Mane

The immune system is our primary line of defense against disease-causing microbes, and a strong immune response is critical for good health. Among its many health benefits, Lion's Mane is known for its immune-boosting properties. This chapter will explore the mechanisms through which Lion's Mane enhances immunity and the implications of this for overall health.

Lion's Mane and Beta-Glucans:

One of the key components responsible for Lion's Mane's immune-enhancing properties is beta-glucans, a type of polysaccharide. Beta-glucans interact with immune cells, including macrophages and natural killer cells, to bolster the body's defenses. They enhance the immune response by stimulating these cells to work more effectively in identifying and neutralizing harmful pathogens.

Modulation of the Immune Response:

Beyond simply stimulating the immune system, Lion's Mane appears to have an immunomodulatory effect. This means it can help balance the immune response, enhancing it when it's underactive (such as in cases of infection) and calming it when it's overactive (as in autoimmune conditions). This regulatory effect can help maintain a healthy immune system and prevent damaging overreactions.

Antioxidant Effects:

Lion's Mane is rich in antioxidants, which can also support the immune system. Oxidative stress can impair immune function, and by neutralizing harmful free radicals, antioxidants help to maintain a healthy immune response. Additionally, antioxidants can protect immune cells from damage, ensuring they're able to function effectively.

Potential Anti-Inflammatory Properties:

Inflammation is a crucial part of the immune response, helping to protect the body against infection and injury. However, when inflammation becomes chronic, it can lead to various health problems. Research suggests that Lion's Mane may have anti-inflammatory properties, potentially helping to reduce unnecessary inflammation and support overall immune health.

Lion's Mane and Gut Health:

The gut plays a crucial role in immunity, housing a significant portion of the body's immune cells. Lion's Mane has been found to promote a healthy gut environment, encouraging the growth of beneficial bacteria and enhancing gut barrier function. These effects can support gut-based immunity and contribute to overall immune health.

In conclusion, Lion's Mane offers numerous immune-boosting benefits. From stimulating immune cells to protecting them from damage and regulating their activity, this unique mushroom can be a valuable addition to an immune-supportive lifestyle. However, it's essential to remember that a strong immune system relies on more than just supplementation – a balanced diet, regular exercise, adequate sleep, and good stress management are all crucial for optimal immune health.

Chapter 8: Lion's Mane and Heart Health

Heart disease is a leading cause of death worldwide, making the search for effective preventative strategies a public health priority. Emerging evidence suggests that Lion's Mane may offer several benefits for heart health, including reducing risk factors for heart disease. This chapter will explore the ways in which Lion's Mane could support heart health.

Lion's Mane and Cholesterol:

High levels of low-density lipoprotein (LDL), or „bad" cholesterol, are a significant risk factor for heart disease. Research suggests that Lion's Mane may help lower LDL levels. In animal studies, the mushroom has been found to reduce total cholesterol and LDL cholesterol levels, potentially reducing the risk of atherosclerosis - the buildup of plaque in the arteries that can lead to heart disease.

Blood Pressure Regulation:

Hypertension, or high blood pressure, is another key risk factor for heart disease. Preliminary research suggests that Lion's Mane may help manage blood pressure levels. While the exact mechanisms aren't fully understood, it's thought that the mushroom's anti-inflammatory and antioxidant effects may contribute to its potential blood pressure-lowering benefits.

Anti-Inflammatory and Antioxidant Effects:

Chronic inflammation and oxidative stress can damage the heart and blood vessels, contributing to heart disease. Lion's Mane contains potent anti-inflammatory and antioxidant compounds that can help reduce inflammation and combat oxidative stress, potentially offering protective benefits for heart health.

Blood Clot Prevention:

Blood clots can lead to serious conditions such as heart attack and stroke. Some research suggests that Lion's Mane may have anticoagulant properties, helping to prevent the formation of dangerous blood clots. However, more research is needed in this area, and it's important to note that people on blood-thinning medications should use Lion's Mane under medical supervision due to potential interactions.

Gut Health and Heart Health:

Emerging research suggests a link between gut health and heart health, with gut imbalances linked to increased heart disease risk. Lion's Mane can support a healthy gut environment, potentially offering indirect benefits for heart health.

In conclusion, while research on Lion's Mane and heart health is still in its early stages, initial findings suggest that the mushroom may offer several heart-protective benefits. From managing heart disease risk factors like high cholesterol and blood pressure to reducing inflammation and oxidative stress,

Lion's Mane could be a valuable addition to a heart-healthy lifestyle. However, it's important to remember that it should not replace conventional heart disease treatments or lifestyle modifications like a balanced diet and regular exercise.

Chapter 9: Anti-Aging Properties of Lion's Mane

Aging is a natural process, but it's often accompanied by a variety of health concerns, from cognitive decline to increased disease risk. Lion's Mane has been touted for its potential anti-aging properties, which are thought to stem from its neuroprotective, antioxidant, and immune-supportive effects. This chapter will explore the potential of Lion's Mane in promoting healthy aging.

Lion's Mane and Cognitive Aging:

As we age, cognitive functions like memory and attention can decline. Lion's Mane's ability to stimulate nerve growth factor production and promote neurogenesis may help counteract this cognitive aging. By supporting neuron health and enhancing cognitive function, Lion's Mane may help maintain cognitive vitality as we age.

Antioxidant Support:

Oxidative stress, caused by an imbalance of free radicals and antioxidants in the body, is believed to be a key factor in aging. By neutralizing harmful free radicals, antioxidants can help protect the body from oxidative damage. Lion's Mane is rich in antioxidants, which may help reduce oxidative stress and its associated aging effects.

Immune Support:

Immune function can decline with age, increasing suscep-tibility to infections and diseases. Lion's Mane's immune-boo-sting properties could help strengthen the immune response in older adults, potentially reducing disease risk and promoting healthier aging.

Anti-Inflammatory Effects:

Chronic inflammation is associated with many aging-related conditions, from heart disease to Alzheimer's. Lion's Mane's potential anti-inflammatory effects could help reduce chronic inflammation, potentially reducing the risk of these conditions and supporting overall health as we age.

Potential Anti-Aging Effects on Skin:

While most of the research on Lion's Mane and aging focuses on internal health, some suggest that the mushroom may also have potential anti-aging benefits for the skin. Its antioxidant properties can protect against oxidative damage, a key cause of skin aging, and its anti-inflammatory effects could help reduce skin inflammation, a contributor to skin conditions like acne and rosacea.

In conclusion, Lion's Mane's potential anti-aging benefits are broad, ranging from cognitive support to skin health. While it's not a magic bullet for aging - a healthy diet, regular exercise, good sleep, and stress management are all crucial for healthy aging - Lion's Mane could be a valuable addition to a holistic approach to aging healthily. As always, it's important to consult with a healthcare provider before starting any new supplement regimen.

Chapter 10: Lion's Mane in Cancer Prevention and Treatment

Cancer remains a major health challenge worldwide, and there is a growing interest in the potential of natural substances, like Lion's Mane, in cancer prevention and treatment. Preclinical studies suggest that Lion's Mane may have anticancer properties, possibly attributed to its immune-enhancing, anti-inflammatory, and antioxidant effects. This chapter will delve into the current understanding of Lion's Mane's potential role in cancer prevention and treatment.

Immune-Enhancing Effects:

Lion's Mane's immune-boosting properties may play a role in cancer prevention and treatment. By enhancing the activity of the immune system, it could potentially help the body recognize and eliminate cancer cells more effectively. Some research suggests that Lion's Mane can stimulate the activity of natural killer cells, a type of immune cell that plays a crucial role in controlling cancer growth.

Anti-Inflammatory and Antioxidant Effects:

Chronic inflammation and oxidative stress are associated with increased cancer risk. Lion's Mane's anti-inflammatory and antioxidant properties could potentially help reduce this risk by reducing inflammation and neutralizing harmful free radicals.

Direct Anticancer Effects:

Beyond its immune, anti-inflammatory, and antioxidant effects, some research suggests that Lion's Mane may have direct anticancer properties. Preclinical studies have found that Lion's Mane extracts can inhibit the growth of various types of cancer cells, including those of the liver, colon, stomach, and blood. However, much more research, particularly in humans, is needed to understand these effects fully.

Lion's Mane and Cancer Symptoms:

Lion's Mane may also help manage some cancer symptoms and treatment side effects. For example, the mushroom has been used traditionally to manage gastric symptoms, which are common in people undergoing cancer treatment. Some evidence also suggests that it may help enhance cognitive function, potentially benefitting people with brain cancer or those experiencing cognitive side effects from cancer treatment.

Considerations and Cautions:

While the potential anticancer effects of Lion's Mane are promising, it's important to note that the mushroom is not a substitute for conventional cancer treatment. It may be used as a complementary approach under the supervision of a healthcare provider, but should not replace standard therapies. Furthermore, people with certain conditions, like mushroom allergies or those taking immunosuppressive drugs, should use Lion's Mane with caution.

In conclusion, Lion's Mane offers promising potential in the realm of cancer prevention and treatment, but much more research is needed to fully understand its therapeutic potential. As always, any use of Lion's Mane in a cancer context should be under the guidance of a healthcare provider.

Chapter 11: Cooking with Lion's Mane: Recipes and Tips

Not only is Lion's Mane mushroom rich in health benefits, but it also offers a unique culinary experience. Its flavor, often likened to seafood like crab or lobster, and its meaty texture make it a versatile ingredient in various dishes. This chapter will provide tips for cooking with Lion's Mane and share some delicious recipes to get you started.

Selecting and Preparing Lion's Mane:

When purchasing fresh Lion's Mane, look for specimens that are clean, firm, and free from blemishes or damp spots. Prior to cooking, clean the mushroom gently with a damp paper towel to remove any dirt or debris. Avoid washing it, as mushrooms are porous and can easily become waterlogged.

Cooking Tips:

Lion's Mane can be sautéed, roasted, grilled, or even fried. When sautéing, cook the mushroom in a bit of oil or butter over medium heat until it's golden brown and slightly crispy. This can take about 10 minutes. For roasting, toss Lion's Mane in a bit of oil, season it with your preferred herbs and spices, and roast it in a preheated oven at 375°F (190°C) until golden brown, around 20-25 minutes.

Lion's Mane „Crab" Cakes Recipe:

Ingredients: 2 cups of shredded Lion's Mane mushroom, 1 cup breadcrumbs, 1/4 cup mayonnaise, 1 egg, 1 teaspoon Dijon mustard, 1 teaspoon Worcestershire sauce, 1/2 teaspoon Old Bay seasoning, salt and pepper to taste, and oil for frying.

Instructions: Mix all the ingredients (except the oil) in a bowl until well combined. Form the mixture into small patties, then fry them in a bit of oil over medium heat until they're golden brown on both sides.

Lion's Mane Pasta Sauce Recipe:

Ingredients: 2 cups of chopped Lion's Mane mushroom, 2 cloves of garlic, 1/2 cup of heavy cream, 1/2 cup of grated Parmesan cheese, salt and pepper to taste, and your favorite pasta.

Instructions: Sauté the Lion's Mane and garlic in a bit of oil until the mushroom is golden brown. Add the cream and simmer until it's reduced by half, then stir in the Parmesan until it's melted and the sauce is creamy. Season with salt and pepper, then toss with your cooked pasta.

Lion's Mane Tea Recipe:

Ingredients: 1 cup of dried Lion's Mane mushroom, 4 cups of water.

Instructions: Combine the dried Lion's Mane and water in a pot, bring it to a boil, then simmer it for about 15 minutes. Strain the tea and enjoy it hot, or cool it down and enjoy it iced.

In conclusion, Lion's Mane is a versatile culinary ingredient that can be used in a variety of dishes. Cooking with Lion's Mane is an excellent way to incorporate this nutritious mushroom into your diet. However, as with any new food, it's important to start with small amounts to see how your body reacts.

Chapter 12: Cultivating Your Own Lion's Mane Mushrooms

Growing your own Lion's Mane mushrooms can be a rewarding and economical way to ensure a steady supply of this superfood. This chapter will guide you through the process of cultivating Lion's Mane mushrooms at home.

Starting from a Kit:

For beginners, starting with a Lion's Mane grow kit can be the easiest option. These kits typically include a block of substrate (the material on which mushrooms grow) that's already inoculated with Lion's Mane spores. To grow the mushrooms, you'll generally need to maintain the right conditions - usually, this involves keeping the kit in a humid, relatively cool place, misting it regularly to maintain moisture, and waiting for the mushrooms to grow.

Starting from Spores:

For a more hands-on (and potentially cost-effective) approach, you can start from Lion's Mane spores. This requires sterilizing a substrate (such as hardwood sawdust), inoculating it with the spores, and maintaining the right conditions for growth. This process requires more effort and equipment than starting from a kit, but it can be a rewarding project for gardening enthusiasts or those interested in mycology.

Caring for Your Lion's Mane:

Regardless of whether you're starting from a kit or spores, caring for your Lion's Mane involves maintaining the right temperature and humidity levels. Lion's Mane prefers temperatures between 60-75°F (15-24°C) and high humidity. Regular misting can help maintain humidity, while keeping the mushrooms out of direct sunlight can help manage temperature.

Harvesting Your Lion's Mane:

You can begin to harvest your Lion's Mane mushrooms once the spines (the long, shaggy pieces that hang down from the mushroom) have fully formed but haven't yet started to turn brown or curl up. To harvest, cut the mushroom off near the base using a sharp knife.

After the Harvest:

After harvesting, the substrate block can often produce another flush (or crop) of mushrooms. Simply continue to care for the block as before, maintaining humidity and temperature, and wait for new mushrooms to grow. After a few flushes, the substrate block will likely be depleted and can be composted.

In conclusion, cultivating your own Lion's Mane mushrooms can be a fun and rewarding project. While it requires some effort and patience, the result is a fresh, homegrown supply of this nutritious and delicious mushroom. As always, ensure to properly identify any homegrown mushrooms before consuming them, and consider seeking guidance from a local mycology expert if you're unsure.

Chapter 13: Risks and Side Effects of Lion's Mane

While Lion's Mane mushroom is generally considered safe for most people when consumed in dietary amounts, it's essential to be aware of potential risks and side effects. This chapter will provide an overview of the known risks and side effects associated with Lion's Mane consumption.

Allergic Reactions:

As with any food or supplement, some individuals may be allergic to Lion's Mane. Signs of an allergic reaction can include itching, rash, difficulty breathing, or swelling of the mouth, face, lips, tongue, or throat. If you experience any of these symptoms after consuming Lion's Mane, you should seek medical attention immediately.

Digestive Upset:

Some people may experience digestive upset, including bloating, gas, or stomach discomfort, when they first start consuming Lion's Mane, particularly in larger amounts or when taken as a supplement. These symptoms typically subside over time as your body adjusts to the new supplement.

Drug Interactions:

Lion's Mane can potentially interact with certain medications. For example, because of its potential effects on blood clotting, it may theoretically increase the risk of bleeding in people taking anticoagulant or antiplatelet drugs. It's always important to discuss any new supplement regimen with a healthcare provider, particularly if you're taking other medications.

Risks for Those with Autoimmune Diseases:

Given its potential to stimulate the immune system, Lion's Mane may theoretically exacerbate symptoms in individuals with autoimmune diseases. If you have an autoimmune condition, you should consult your healthcare provider before starting Lion's Mane.

Risks of Contamination:

When purchasing Lion's Mane, whether fresh or as a supplement, it's important to choose products from reputable sources. Some mushrooms can absorb and accumulate heavy metals from their environment, which can be harmful if ingested.

In conclusion, while Lion's Mane is generally considered safe for most people, it's important to be aware of potential risks and side effects. As with any new food or supplement, it's always best to start with small amounts to see how your body reacts and to discuss any new supplement regimen with a healthcare provider.

Chapter 14: Lion's Mane in Traditional and Modern Medicine

Lion's Mane mushroom has a rich history in traditional medicine and is now being recognized in modern medicine for its potential health benefits. This chapter will explore Lion's Mane's role in both traditional and modern medical practices.

Lion's Mane in Traditional Medicine:

Lion's Mane has been used in traditional Chinese and Japanese medicine for centuries. It was often consumed as a general health tonic and used to treat a variety of conditions, including digestive and neurological disorders. Traditional healers prized Lion's Mane for its ability to improve digestion, boost cognitive function, and strengthen the nervous system.

Lion's Mane in Modern Medicine:

Modern medicine is beginning to recognize the potential health benefits of Lion's Mane, with several studies exploring its medicinal properties. The mushroom's potential effects on neurological health have been a particular focus, with research suggesting that it may help support cognitive function, prevent neurodegenerative diseases, and promote nerve regeneration. Additionally, studies have examined Lion's Mane's potential anticancer, immune-boosting, and anti-inflammatory properties.

The Science Behind Lion's Mane:

Much of Lion's Mane's potential medicinal properties are believed to stem from its unique compounds, including hericenones and erinacines, which can stimulate the production of nerve growth factor, a protein that plays a crucial role in maintaining and repairing neurons. Lion's Mane also contains potent antioxidants and beta-glucans, which may contribute to its immune-boosting and anti-inflammatory effects.

Lion's Mane as a Dietary Supplement:

Given its potential health benefits, Lion's Mane is widely available as a dietary supplement. These supplements come in various forms, including capsules, powders, and tinctures, and are often used for their potential cognitive-enhancing and immune-boosting effects.

Future Research:

While the current research on Lion's Mane is promising, more extensive clinical trials are needed to fully understand its therapeutic potential and to establish standardized dosages and protocols for its use. Future research will likely continue to explore Lion's Mane's potential neurological benefits, along with its potential roles in cancer prevention, immune support, and more.

In conclusion, Lion's Mane holds a special place in both traditional and modern medicine. Its potential health benefits, combined with its culinary versatility, make it a unique and promising functional food and supplement. As always, it's important to consult with a healthcare provider before starting any new supplement regimen.

Chapter 15: The Future of Lion's Mane: Research and Possibilities

The Lion's Mane mushroom, having already established its position in traditional medicine and having shown promising potential in modern research, looks toward a future ripe with possibilities. This chapter will delve into the future research directions and potential applications of Lion's Mane.

Continued Research in Neurological Health:

Given the promising preliminary results on the benefits of Lion's Mane on neurological health, researchers will likely continue exploring its potential effects on cognitive function, neurodegenerative diseases, and nerve repair. Future research could provide more definitive evidence of its efficacy and guide the development of new therapies for various neurological conditions.

Potential in Cancer Treatment:

Early studies have indicated that Lion's Mane may have anticancer properties. Its beta-glucan compounds appear to inhibit the growth of certain cancer cells. Future research may delve deeper into these potential anticancer properties, exploring how they can be harnessed in cancer treatment or prevention.

Immune System Research:

The immune-boosting properties of Lion's Mane, attributed to its high antioxidant content, will likely be another focal point for future research. Understanding how Lion's Mane interacts with our immune system could lead to innovative strategies for enhancing immune function and combating diseases.

Exploration of Other Health Benefits:

While current research has focused primarily on Lion's Mane's neurological, immune, and anticancer benefits, future studies may uncover other health benefits. For instance, Lion's Mane's potential effects on gut health, heart health, and overall longevity could be explored further.

Sustainable Cultivation Practices:

As the popularity of Lion's Mane continues to grow, ensuring sustainable cultivation practices will become increasingly important. Research into optimizing growth conditions and developing eco-friendly cultivation methods will play a critical role in ensuring a sustainable supply of Lion's Mane.

Broadening Accessibility:

Efforts to make Lion's Mane more accessible will likely continue. This could involve developing more affordable Lion's Mane supplements or initiatives to educate the public about how to grow their own Lion's Mane mushrooms at home.

In conclusion, the future of Lion's Mane looks promising. With continued research, improved cultivation practices, and efforts to broaden its accessibility, this unique mushroom will likely continue to grow in popularity as a functional food and supplement. The potential health benefits of Lion's Mane could transform it into a key player in the future of integrative and preventive medicine.

Disclaimer

This book is intended to provide general information about Lion's Mane mushroom, its history, cultivation, potential health benefits, and uses in cooking. The content is not intended to replace professional medical advice, diagnosis, or treatment. Always seek the advice of your healthcare provider or a qualified health professional with any questions you may have regarding a medical condition.

Never disregard professional medical advice or delay in seeking it because of something you have read in this book. If you think you may have a medical emergency, call your doctor or emergency services immediately.

The information contained herein is based on research available up to the publication date. As research progresses, some information may become outdated.

While every effort has been made to ensure that the information provided in this book is accurate and up-to-date at the time of publication, the author and publisher make no representations or warranties of any kind, express or implied, about the completeness, accuracy, reliability, suitability, or availability concerning the book or the information, products, services, or related graphics contained in the book for any purpose.

The author and publisher are not responsible for any errors or omissions or for the results obtained from the use of this information. All information in this book is provided „as is" with no guarantee of completeness, accuracy, timeliness, or of the results obtained from the use of this information, and without warranty of any kind, express or implied.

Your use of this book is strictly at your own risk. In no event will the author or publisher be liable for any loss or damage including without limitation, indirect or consequential loss or damage, or any loss or damage whatsoever arising from loss of data or profits arising out of, or in connection with, the use of this book.

List with different names of the mushroom:

Country/Region	Name in Local Language	Translation
China	猴头菇 (Hóutóu gū)	Monkey Head Mushroom
Japan	ヤマブシタケ (Yamabushitake)	Yamabushi Mushroom
Korea	노란영지 (Nolan yeongji)	Yellow Mushroom
Russia	Гриб Левины гривы (Grib Leviny grivy)	Lion's Mane Mushroom
Germany	Igel-Stachelbart	Hedgehog Goatee
France	Hydne hérisson	Hedgehog Hydnum
Spain	Melena de león	Lion's Mane
Italy	Criniera di leone	Lion's Mane

Other books by the author

Neanderthals: Unraveling the Secrets of Our Ancient Relatives

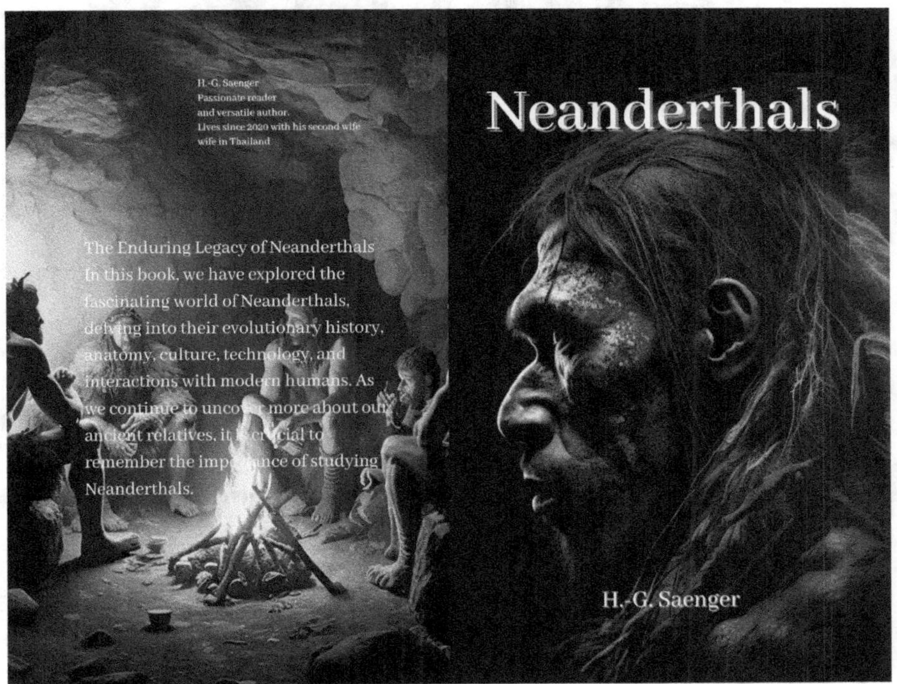

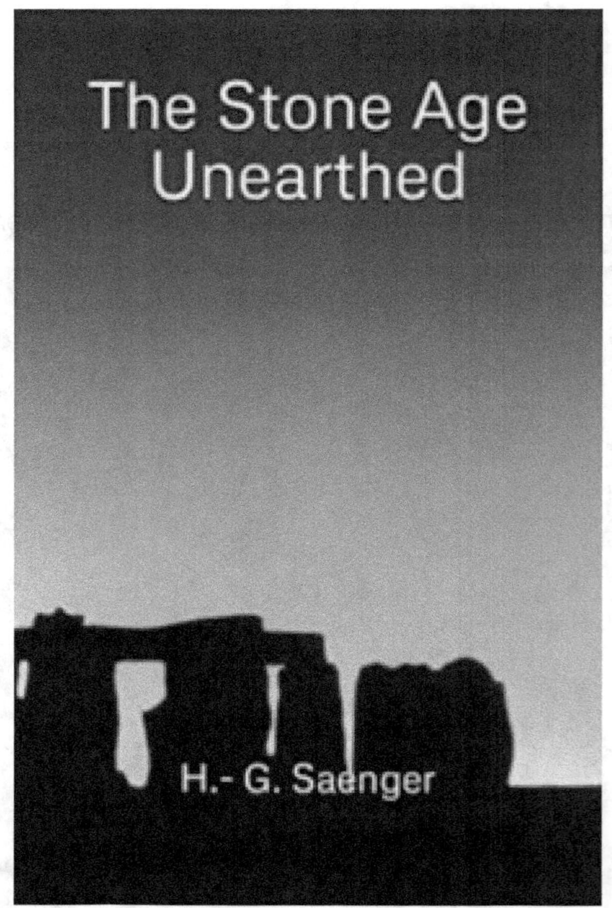

The Stone Age
Unearthed
H.- G. Saenger

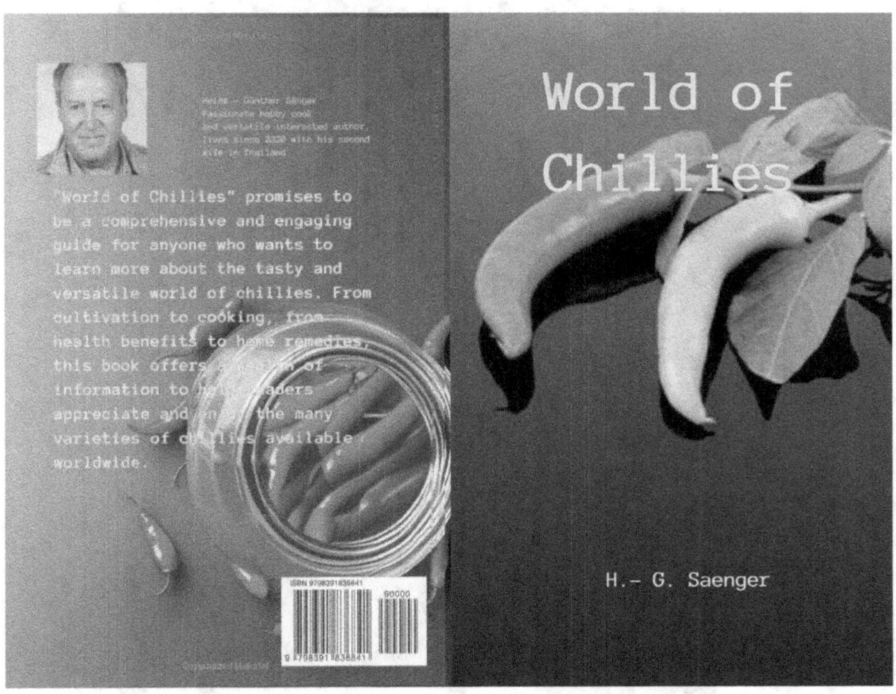
World of
Chillies

"World of Chillies" promises to
be a comprehensive and engaging
guide for anyone who wants to
learn more about the tasty and
versatile world of chillies. From
cultivation to cooking, from
health benefits to home remedies,
this book offers a wealth of
information to help readers
appreciate and enjoy the many
varieties of chillies available
worldwide.

H.- G. Saenger

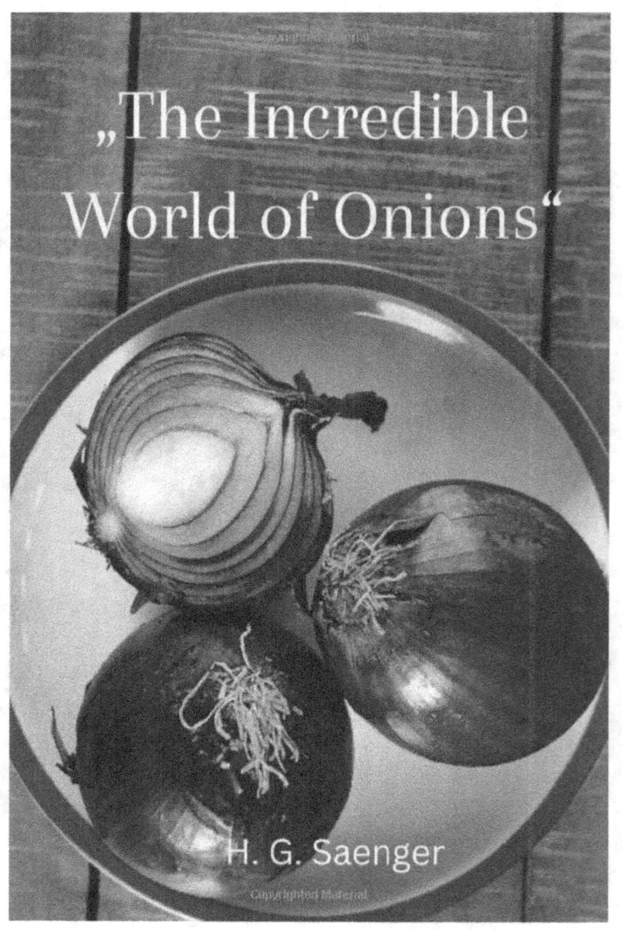
„The Incredible
World of Onions"
H. G. Saenger

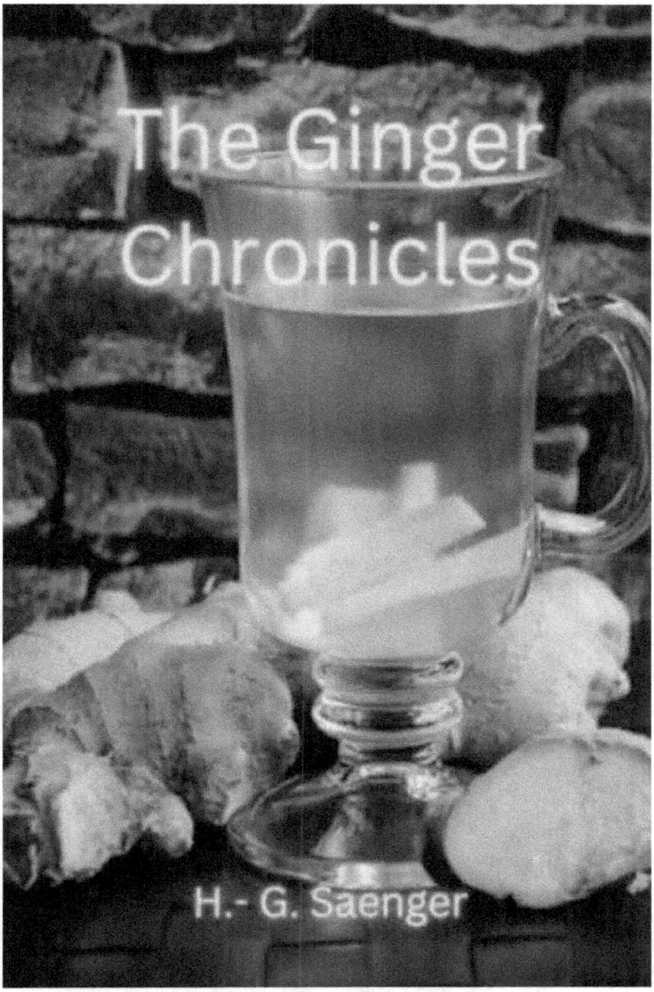

H.-G. Saenger

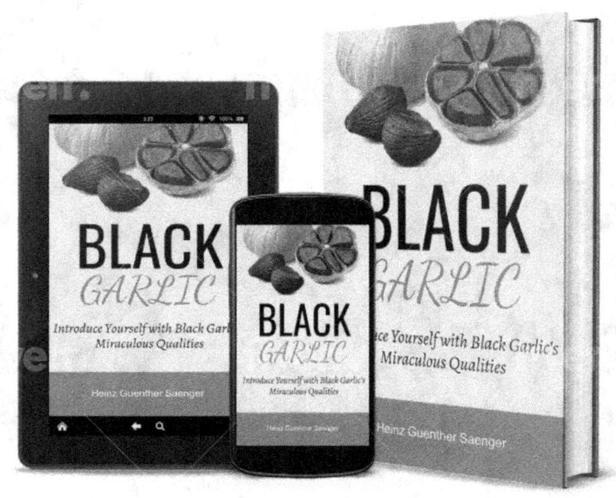

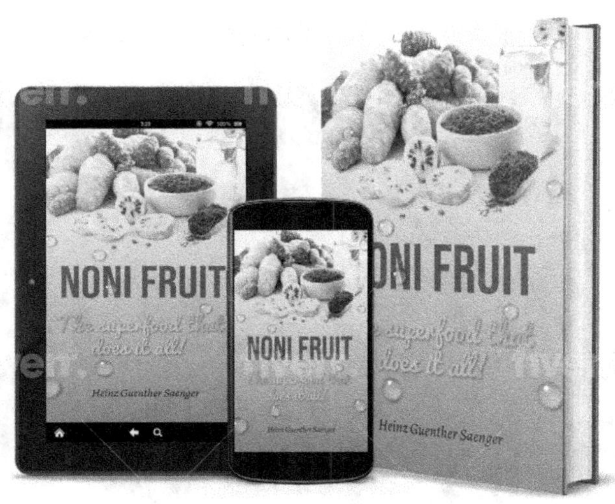
NONI FRUIT
The superfood that does it all!
Heinz Guenther Saenger
NONI FRUIT
The superfood that does it all!
Heinz Guenther Saenger

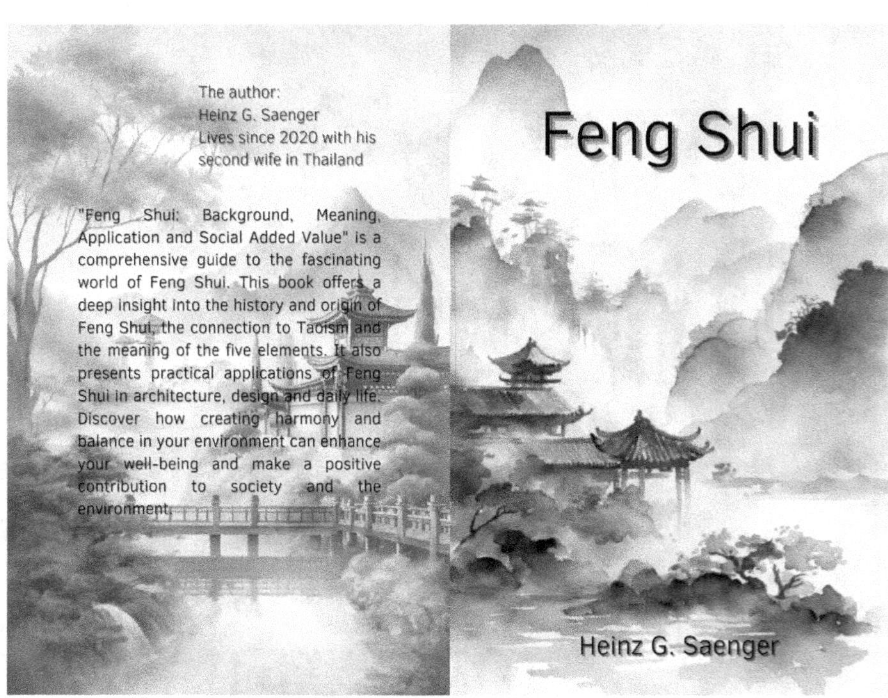

The author:
Heinz G. Saenger
Lives since 2020 with his
second wife in Thailand

"Feng Shui: Background, Meaning,
Application and Social Added Value" is a
comprehensive guide to the fascinating
world of Feng Shui. This book offers a
deep insight into the history and origin of
Feng Shui, the connection to Taoism and
the meaning of the five elements. It also
presents practical applications of Feng
Shui in architecture, design and daily life.
Discover how creating harmony and
balance in your environment can enhance
your well-being and make a positive
contribution to society and the
environment.

Feng Shui

Heinz G. Saenger

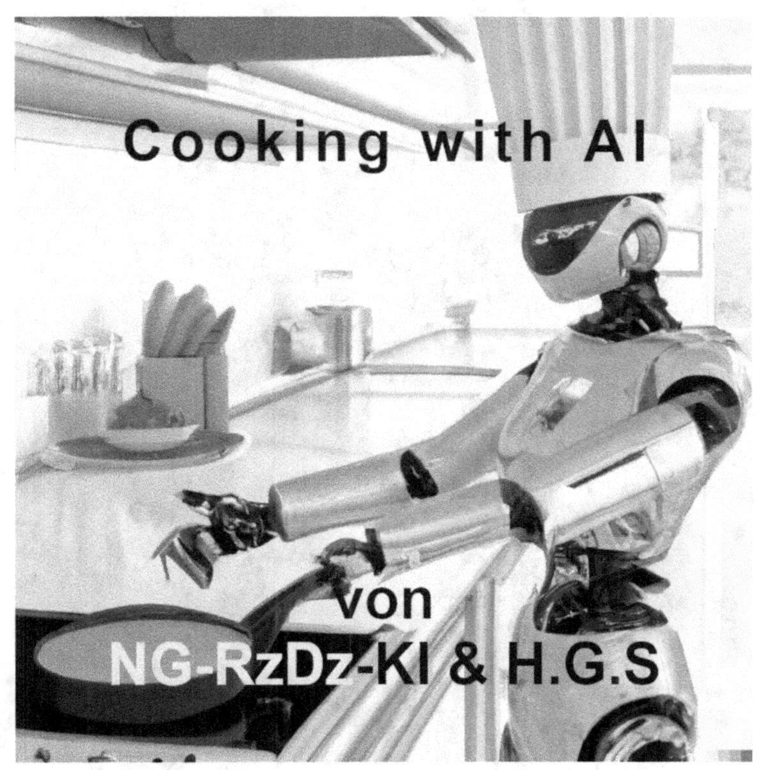
Cooking with AI
von
NG-RzDz-KI & H.G.S

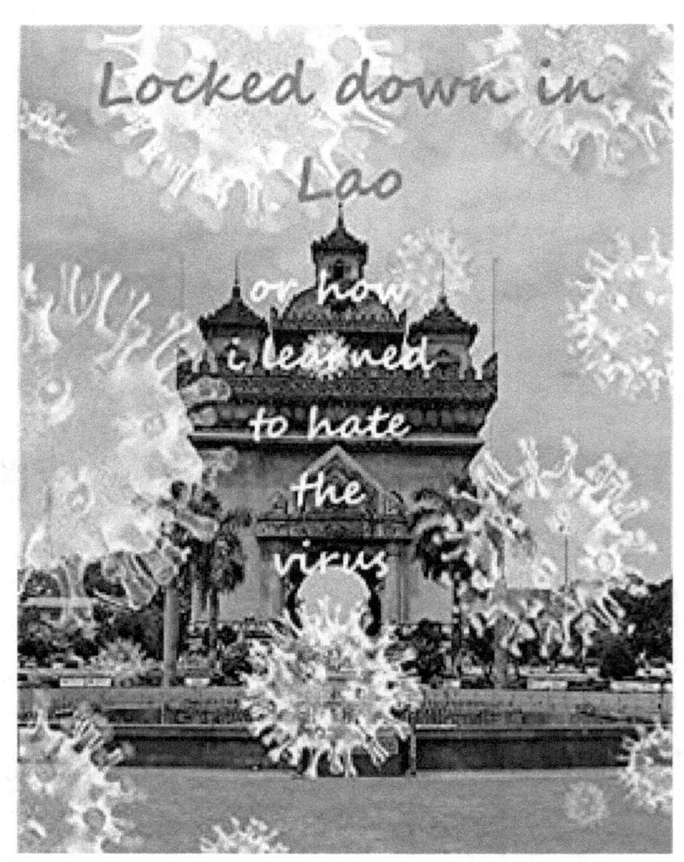

Locked down in
Lao
or how
i learned
to hate
the
virus

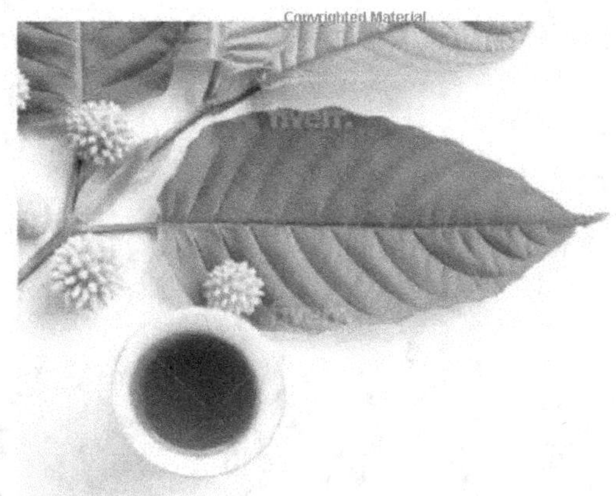

KRATOM FOR NEWBIES

All You Need To Know About Kratom Usage

By Heinz Guenther Saenger

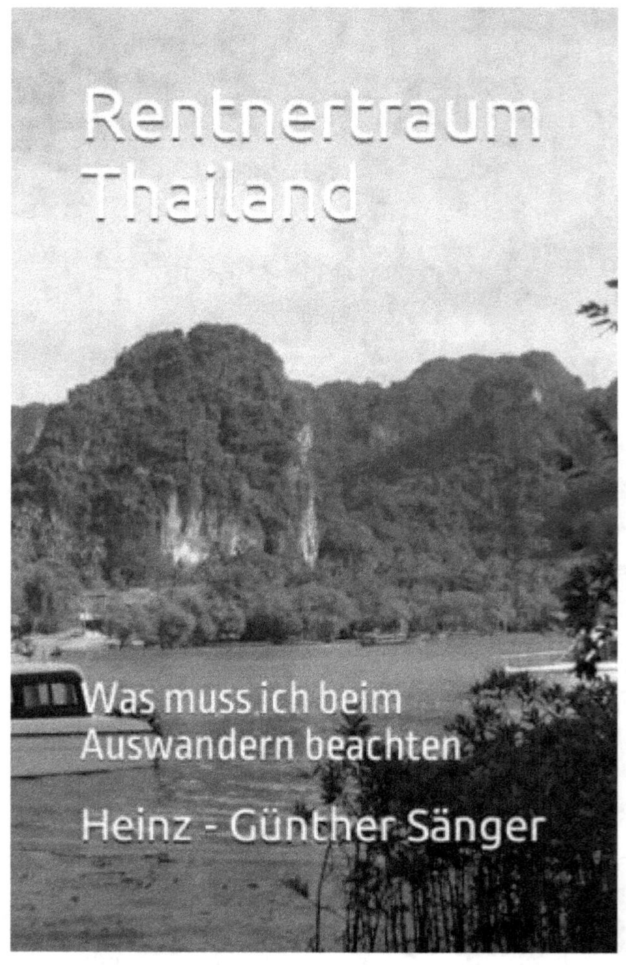
Rentnertraum
Thailand
Was muss ich beim
Auswandern beachten
Heinz - Günther Sänger

H.-G. Saenger

Turmeric: The Golden Treasure of Asia

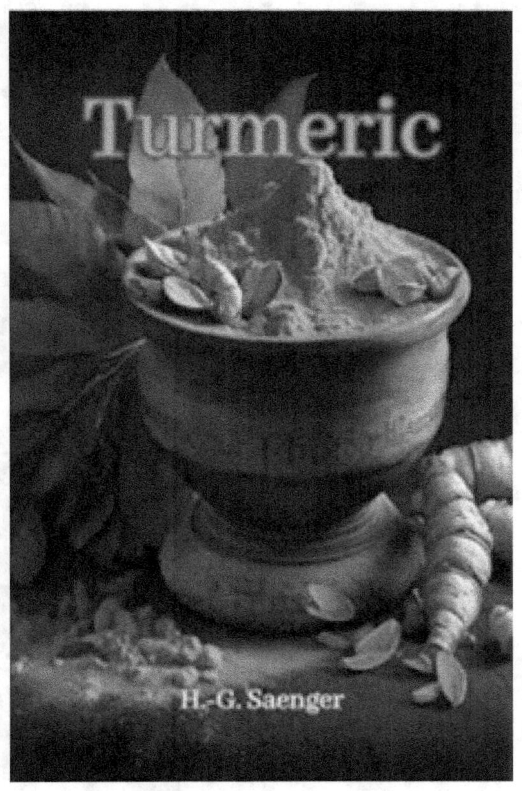

Turmeric: The Golden Treasure of Asia

Coconut: The remarkable world of the coconut

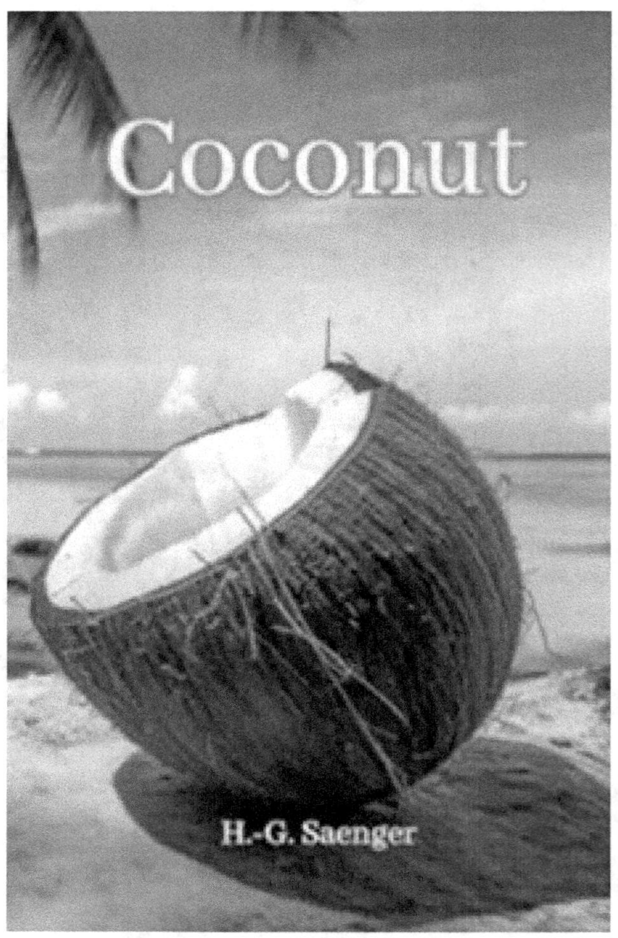

www.ingramcontent.com/pod-product-compliance
Lightning Source LLC
Chambersburg PA
CBHW051844250726
48659CB00005B/2016